THIS PLANNER BELONGS TO :

DAILY PLANNER

DATE: ———————— DAY: ————————

TO DO LIST

- [ ] ________________________
- [ ] ________________________
- [ ] ________________________
- [ ] ________________________
- [ ] ________________________
- [ ] ________________________
- [ ] ________________________

PERSONAL NOTES

TOP PRIORITIES

- [ ] ________________________
- [ ] ________________________

- [ ] ________________________
- [ ] ________________________

APPOINTMENTS & EVENTS

GET IN TOUCH WITH

- [ ] ________________________
- [ ] ________________________

MEALS

Breakfast

Lunch

Dinner

DAILY PLANNER

DATE: ________________ DAY: ________________

TO DO LIST

- [ ]
- [ ]
- [ ]
- [ ]
- [ ]
- [ ]
- [ ]

PERSONAL NOTES

TOP PRIORITIES

- [ ]
- [ ]

- [ ]
- [ ]

APPOINTMENTS & EVENTS

GET IN TOUCH WITH

- [ ]
- [ ]

MEALS

Breakfast

Lunch

Dinner

DAILY PLANNER

DATE: _______________   DAY: _______________

TO DO LIST

PERSONAL NOTES

TOP PRIORITIES

APPOINTMENTS & EVENTS

GET IN TOUCH WITH

MEALS

Breakfast

Lunch

Dinner

DAILY PLANNER

DATE: _______________ DAY: _______________

TO DO LIST

- ☐ _______________
- ☐ _______________
- ☐ _______________
- ☐ _______________
- ☐ _______________
- ☐ _______________
- ☐ _______________

PERSONAL NOTES

TOP PRIORITIES

- ☐ _______________
- ☐ _______________

- ☐ _______________
- ☐ _______________

APPOINTMENTS & EVENTS

GET IN TOUCH WITH

- ☐ _______________
- ☐ _______________

MEALS

Breakfast

Lunch

Dinner

DAILY PLANNER

DATE: _______________ DAY: _______________

TO DO LIST

- [ ] _______________
- [ ] _______________
- [ ] _______________
- [ ] _______________
- [ ] _______________
- [ ] _______________
- [ ] _______________

PERSONAL NOTES

TOP PRIORITIES

- [ ] _______________
- [ ] _______________

APPOINTMENTS & EVENTS

GET IN TOUCH WITH

- [ ] _______________
- [ ] _______________

MEALS

Breakfast

Lunch

Dinner

DAILY PLANNER

DATE: ——————   DAY: ——————

TO DO LIST

- ☐ ____________________
- ☐ ____________________
- ☐ ____________________
- ☐ ____________________
- ☐ ____________________
- ☐ ____________________
- ☐ ____________________

PERSONAL NOTES

TOP PRIORITIES

- ☐ ____________________
- ☐ ____________________
- ☐ ____________________
- ☐ ____________________

APPOINTMENTS & EVENTS

GET IN TOUCH WITH

- ☐ ____________________
- ☐ ____________________

MEALS

Breakfast

Lunch

Dinner

DAILY PLANNER

DATE: ___________ DAY: ___________

TO DO LIST

- ☐ _______________________
- ☐ _______________________
- ☐ _______________________
- ☐ _______________________
- ☐ _______________________
- ☐ _______________________
- ☐ _______________________

PERSONAL NOTES

TOP PRIORITIES

- ☐ _______________________
- ☐ _______________________
- ☐ _______________________
- ☐ _______________________

APPOINTMENTS & EVENTS

GET IN TOUCH WITH

- ☐ _______________________
- ☐ _______________________

MEALS

Breakfast

Lunch

Dinner

WEEKLY PLANNER

MONTH:

MONDAY

TUESDAY

WEDNESDAY

THURSDAY

FRIDAY

SATURDAY

SUNDAY

TO DO LIST

HABITS TRACKER

M T W T F S S

PERSONAL NOTES

MEAL PLANNER

WEEK: ——————— MONTH: ———————

MONDAY

B
L
D
S

TUESDAY

B
L
D
S

WEDNESDAY

B
L
D
S

THURSDAY

B
L
D
S

FRIDAY

B
L
D
S

SATURDAY

B
L
D
S

SUNDAY

B
L
D
S

THIS WEEK'S GROCERY LIST

- [ ]
- [ ]
- [ ]
- [ ]
- [ ]
- [ ]
- [ ]
- [ ]
- [ ]
- [ ]
- [ ]
- [ ]
- [ ]
- [ ]
- [ ]
- [ ]
- [ ]

THIS WEEK'S GROCERY LIST

DAILY PLANNER

DATE: ——————— DAY: ———————

TO DO LIST

PERSONAL NOTES

TOP PRIORITIES

APPOINTMENTS & EVENTS

GET IN TOUCH WITH

MEALS

Breakfast

Lunch

Dinner

DAILY PLANNER

DATE: ___________   DAY: ___________

TO DO LIST

- [ ] ___________
- [ ] ___________
- [ ] ___________
- [ ] ___________
- [ ] ___________
- [ ] ___________
- [ ] ___________

PERSONAL NOTES

TOP PRIORITIES

- [ ] ___________
- [ ] ___________

- [ ] ___________
- [ ] ___________

APPOINTMENTS & EVENTS

GET IN TOUCH WITH

- [ ] ___________
- [ ] ___________

MEALS

Breakfast

Lunch

Dinner

DAILY PLANNER

DATE: —————— DAY: ——————

TO DO LIST

PERSONAL NOTES

TOP PRIORITIES

APPOINTMENTS & EVENTS

GET IN TOUCH WITH

MEALS

Breakfast

Lunch

Dinner

DAILY PLANNER

DATE: ____________ DAY: ____________

TO DO LIST

- ☐ ___________________________
- ☐ ___________________________
- ☐ ___________________________
- ☐ ___________________________
- ☐ ___________________________
- ☐ ___________________________
- ☐ ___________________________

PERSONAL NOTES

TOP PRIORITIES

- ☐ ___________________________
- ☐ ___________________________

- ☐ ___________________________
- ☐ ___________________________

APPOINTMENTS & EVENTS

GET IN TOUCH WITH

- ☐ ___________________________
- ☐ ___________________________

MEALS

Breakfast

Lunch

Dinner

DAILY PLANNER

DATE: _______________   DAY: _______________

TO DO LIST

- ☐ _______________
- ☐ _______________
- ☐ _______________
- ☐ _______________
- ☐ _______________
- ☐ _______________
- ☐ _______________

PERSONAL NOTES

TOP PRIORITIES

- ☐ _______________
- ☐ _______________

- ☐ _______________
- ☐ _______________

APPOINTMENTS & EVENTS

GET IN TOUCH WITH

- ☐ _______________
- ☐ _______________

MEALS

Breakfast

Lunch

Dinner

DAILY PLANNER

DATE: ______________ DAY: ______________

TO DO LIST

- ☐ ____________________
- ☐ ____________________
- ☐ ____________________
- ☐ ____________________
- ☐ ____________________
- ☐ ____________________
- ☐ ____________________

PERSONAL NOTES

TOP PRIORITIES

- ☐ ____________________
- ☐ ____________________

- ☐ ____________________
- ☐ ____________________

APPOINTMENTS & EVENTS

GET IN TOUCH WITH

- ☐ ____________________
- ☐ ____________________

MEALS

Breakfast

Lunch

Dinner

DAILY PLANNER

DATE: _______________ DAY: _______________

TO DO LIST

☐ _______________
☐ _______________
☐ _______________
☐ _______________
☐ _______________
☐ _______________
☐ _______________

TOP PRIORITIES

☐ _______________   ☐ _______________
☐ _______________   ☐ _______________

APPOINTMENTS & EVENTS

PERSONAL NOTES

GET IN TOUCH WITH

☐ _______________
☐ _______________

MEALS

Breakfast

Lunch

Dinner

WEEKLY PLANNER

MONTH: _______________

MONDAY

TUESDAY

WEDNESDAY

THURSDAY

FRIDAY

SATURDAY

SUNDAY

TO DO LIST

- ☐ _______________
- ☐ _______________
- ☐ _______________
- ☐ _______________
- ☐ _______________
- ☐ _______________
- ☐ _______________

HABITS TRACKER

M T W T F S S

PERSONAL NOTES

MEAL PLANNER

WEEK: _________ MONTH: _________

MONDAY

B ___________________________
L ___________________________
D ___________________________
S ___________________________

TUESDAY

B ___________________________
L ___________________________
D ___________________________
S ___________________________

WEDNESDAY

B ___________________________
L ___________________________
D ___________________________
S ___________________________

THURSDAY

B ___________________________
L ___________________________
D ___________________________
S ___________________________

FRIDAY

B ___________________________
L ___________________________
D ___________________________
S ___________________________

SATURDAY

B ___________________________
L ___________________________
D ___________________________
S ___________________________

SUNDAY

B ___________________________
L ___________________________
D ___________________________
S ___________________________

THIS WEEK'S GROCERY LIST

☐ ___________________________
☐ ___________________________
☐ ___________________________
☐ ___________________________
☐ ___________________________
☐ ___________________________
☐ ___________________________
☐ ___________________________
☐ ___________________________
☐ ___________________________
☐ ___________________________
☐ ___________________________
☐ ___________________________
☐ ___________________________
☐ ___________________________
☐ ___________________________
☐ ___________________________

DAILY PLANNER

DATE: _____________ DAY: _____________

TO DO LIST

PERSONAL NOTES

TOP PRIORITIES

APPOINTMENTS & EVENTS

GET IN TOUCH WITH

MEALS

Breakfast

Lunch

Dinner

DAILY PLANNER

DATE: ________________ DAY: ________________

TO DO LIST

- [ ] ___________________________
- [ ] ___________________________
- [ ] ___________________________
- [ ] ___________________________
- [ ] ___________________________
- [ ] ___________________________
- [ ] ___________________________

PERSONAL NOTES

TOP PRIORITIES

- [ ] ___________________________
- [ ] ___________________________

- [ ] ___________________________
- [ ] ___________________________

APPOINTMENTS & EVENTS

GET IN TOUCH WITH

- [ ] ___________________________
- [ ] ___________________________

MEALS

Breakfast

Lunch

Dinner

DAILY PLANNER

DATE: ______________   DAY: ______________

TO DO LIST

- ☐ ___________________
- ☐ ___________________
- ☐ ___________________
- ☐ ___________________
- ☐ ___________________
- ☐ ___________________
- ☐ ___________________

PERSONAL NOTES

TOP PRIORITIES

- ☐ ___________________
- ☐ ___________________

- ☐ ___________________
- ☐ ___________________

APPOINTMENTS & EVENTS

GET IN TOUCH WITH

- ☐ ___________________
- ☐ ___________________

MEALS

Breakfast

Lunch

Dinner

DAILY PLANNER

DATE: —————— DAY: ——————

TO DO LIST

- [ ]
- [ ]
- [ ]
- [ ]
- [ ]
- [ ]
- [ ]

PERSONAL NOTES

TOP PRIORITIES

- [ ]
- [ ]

- [ ]
- [ ]

APPOINTMENTS & EVENTS

GET IN TOUCH WITH

- [ ]
- [ ]

MEALS

Breakfast

Lunch

Dinner

DAILY PLANNER

DATE: ___________ DAY: ___________

TO DO LIST

- [ ] _______________
- [ ] _______________
- [ ] _______________
- [ ] _______________
- [ ] _______________
- [ ] _______________
- [ ] _______________

PERSONAL NOTES

TOP PRIORITIES

- [ ] _______________
- [ ] _______________
- [ ] _______________
- [ ] _______________

APPOINTMENTS & EVENTS

GET IN TOUCH WITH

- [ ] _______________
- [ ] _______________

MEALS

Breakfast

Lunch

Dinner

DAILY PLANNER

DATE: __________ DAY: __________

TO DO LIST

- ☐ _______________________
- ☐ _______________________
- ☐ _______________________
- ☐ _______________________
- ☐ _______________________
- ☐ _______________________
- ☐ _______________________

PERSONAL NOTES

TOP PRIORITIES

- ☐ _______________________
- ☐ _______________________

- ☐ _______________________
- ☐ _______________________

APPOINTMENTS & EVENTS

GET IN TOUCH WITH

- ☐ _______________________
- ☐ _______________________

MEALS

Breakfast

Lunch

Dinner

DAILY PLANNER

DATE: —————— DAY: ——————

TO DO LIST

- ☐ ______________________
- ☐ ______________________
- ☐ ______________________
- ☐ ______________________
- ☐ ______________________
- ☐ ______________________
- ☐ ______________________

PERSONAL NOTES

TOP PRIORITIES

- ☐ ______________________
- ☐ ______________________

- ☐ ______________________
- ☐ ______________________

APPOINTMENTS & EVENTS

GET IN TOUCH WITH

- ☐ ______________________
- ☐ ______________________

MEALS

Breakfast

Lunch

Dinner

WEEKLY PLANNER

MONTH: ___________________

MONDAY

TUESDAY

WEDNESDAY

THURSDAY

FRIDAY

SATURDAY

SUNDAY

TO DO LIST

- [ ]
- [ ]
- [ ]
- [ ]
- [ ]
- [ ]
- [ ]

HABITS TRACKER

M T W T F S S

PERSONAL NOTES

MEAL PLANNER

WEEK: ________   MONTH: ________

MONDAY

B
L
D
S

TUESDAY

B
L
D
S

WEDNESDAY

B
L
D
S

THURSDAY

B
L
D
S

FRIDAY

B
L
D
S

SATURDAY

B
L
D
S

SUNDAY

B
L
D
S

THIS WEEK'S GROCERY LIST

- [ ]
- [ ]
- [ ]
- [ ]
- [ ]
- [ ]
- [ ]
- [ ]
- [ ]
- [ ]
- [ ]
- [ ]
- [ ]
- [ ]
- [ ]
- [ ]
- [ ]

DAILY PLANNER

DATE: ———————   DAY: ———————

TO DO LIST

- ☐ ______________________
- ☐ ______________________
- ☐ ______________________
- ☐ ______________________
- ☐ ______________________
- ☐ ______________________
- ☐ ______________________

PERSONAL NOTES

TOP PRIORITIES

- ☐ ______________________
- ☐ ______________________

- ☐ ______________________
- ☐ ______________________

APPOINTMENTS & EVENTS

GET IN TOUCH WITH

- ☐ ______________________
- ☐ ______________________

MEALS

Breakfast

Lunch

Dinner

DAILY PLANNER

DATE: _______________ DAY: _______________

TO DO LIST

☐ _______________
☐ _______________
☐ _______________
☐ _______________
☐ _______________
☐ _______________
☐ _______________

PERSONAL NOTES

TOP PRIORITIES

☐ _______________   ☐ _______________
☐ _______________   ☐ _______________

APPOINTMENTS & EVENTS

GET IN TOUCH WITH

☐ _______________
☐ _______________

MEALS

Breakfast

Lunch

Dinner

DAILY PLANNER

DATE: _______________ DAY: _______________

TO DO LIST

- [ ] _______________
- [ ] _______________
- [ ] _______________
- [ ] _______________
- [ ] _______________
- [ ] _______________
- [ ] _______________

TOP PRIORITIES

- [ ] _______________
- [ ] _______________
- [ ] _______________
- [ ] _______________

APPOINTMENTS & EVENTS

PERSONAL NOTES

GET IN TOUCH WITH

- [ ] _______________
- [ ] _______________

MEALS

Breakfast

Lunch

Dinner

DAILY PLANNER

DATE: _____________ DAY: _____________

TO DO LIST

- [ ] _____________________________
- [ ] _____________________________
- [ ] _____________________________
- [ ] _____________________________
- [ ] _____________________________
- [ ] _____________________________
- [ ] _____________________________

PERSONAL NOTES

TOP PRIORITIES

- [ ] _____________________________
- [ ] _____________________________
- [ ] _____________________________
- [ ] _____________________________

APPOINTMENTS & EVENTS

GET IN TOUCH WITH

- [ ] _____________________________
- [ ] _____________________________

MEALS

Breakfast

Lunch

Dinner

DAILY PLANNER

DATE: ———— DAY: ————

TO DO LIST

- ☐ ______________________
- ☐ ______________________
- ☐ ______________________
- ☐ ______________________
- ☐ ______________________
- ☐ ______________________
- ☐ ______________________

PERSONAL NOTES

TOP PRIORITIES

- ☐ ______________________
- ☐ ______________________

- ☐ ______________________
- ☐ ______________________

APPOINTMENTS & EVENTS

GET IN TOUCH WITH

- ☐ ______________________
- ☐ ______________________

MEALS

Breakfast

Lunch

Dinner

DAILY PLANNER

DATE: ——————— DAY: ———————

TO DO LIST

PERSONAL NOTES

TOP PRIORITIES

APPOINTMENTS & EVENTS

GET IN TOUCH WITH

MEALS

Breakfast

Lunch

Dinner

DAILY PLANNER

DATE: —————— DAY: ——————

TO DO LIST

- [ ]
- [ ]
- [ ]
- [ ]
- [ ]
- [ ]
- [ ]

PERSONAL NOTES

TOP PRIORITIES

- [ ]
- [ ]

- [ ]
- [ ]

APPOINTMENTS & EVENTS

GET IN TOUCH WITH

- [ ]
- [ ]

MEALS

Breakfast

Lunch

Dinner

WEEKLY PLANNER

MONTH:

MONDAY

TUESDAY

WEDNESDAY

THURSDAY

FRIDAY

SATURDAY

SUNDAY

TO DO LIST

HABITS TRACKER

M T W T F S S

PERSONAL NOTES

MEAL PLANNER

WEEK: ———————— MONTH: ————————

MONDAY
B
L
D
S

TUESDAY
B
L
D
S

WEDNESDAY
B
L
D
S

THURSDAY
B
L
D
S

FRIDAY
B
L
D
S

SATURDAY
B
L
D
S

SUNDAY
B
L
D
S

THIS WEEK'S GROCERY LIST

THIS WEEK'S GROCERY LIST

FITNESS TRACKER

MONTH: ______

WEIGHT

105KG
95KG
85KG
75KG
65KG
55KG
45KG
35KG

JAN FEB MAR APR MAY JUN JUL AUG SEP OCT NOV DEC

MEASUREMENTS

	BUST	WAIST	HIPS	BUTT
JAN				
FEB				
MAR				
APR				
MAY				
JUN				
JUL				
AUG				
SEP				
OCT				
NOV				
DEC				

READING TRACKER

MONTH:

TITLE	AUTHOR	GENRE	RATING
			☆ ☆ ☆ ☆ ☆
			☆ ☆ ☆ ☆ ☆
			☆ ☆ ☆ ☆ ☆
			☆ ☆ ☆ ☆ ☆
			☆ ☆ ☆ ☆ ☆
			☆ ☆ ☆ ☆ ☆
			☆ ☆ ☆ ☆ ☆
			☆ ☆ ☆ ☆ ☆
			☆ ☆ ☆ ☆ ☆
			☆ ☆ ☆ ☆ ☆
			☆ ☆ ☆ ☆ ☆
			☆ ☆ ☆ ☆ ☆

DAILY PLANNER

DATE: ________________ DAY: ________________

TO DO LIST

PERSONAL NOTES

TOP PRIORITIES

APPOINTMENTS & EVENTS

GET IN TOUCH WITH

MEALS

Breakfast

Lunch

Dinner

DAILY PLANNER

DATE: ———————— DAY: ————————

TO DO LIST

PERSONAL NOTES

TOP PRIORITIES

APPOINTMENTS & EVENTS

GET IN TOUCH WITH

MEALS

Breakfast

Lunch

Dinner

DAILY PLANNER

DATE: ————— DAY: —————

TO DO LIST

PERSONAL NOTES

TOP PRIORITIES

APPOINTMENTS & EVENTS

GET IN TOUCH WITH

MEALS

Breakfast

Lunch

Dinner

DAILY PLANNER

DATE: __________ DAY: __________

TO DO LIST

PERSONAL NOTES

TOP PRIORITIES

APPOINTMENTS & EVENTS

GET IN TOUCH WITH

MEALS

Breakfast

Lunch

Dinner

DAILY PLANNER

DATE: __________ DAY: __________

TO DO LIST

PERSONAL NOTES

TOP PRIORITIES

APPOINTMENTS & EVENTS

GET IN TOUCH WITH

MEALS

Breakfast

Lunch

Dinner

DAILY PLANNER

DATE: _______________ DAY: _______________

TO DO LIST

PERSONAL NOTES

TOP PRIORITIES

APPOINTMENTS & EVENTS

GET IN TOUCH WITH

MEALS

Breakfast

Lunch

Dinner

DAILY PLANNER

DATE: _______________ DAY: _______________

TO DO LIST

- [ ] ___________________
- [ ] ___________________
- [ ] ___________________
- [ ] ___________________
- [ ] ___________________
- [ ] ___________________
- [ ] ___________________

PERSONAL NOTES

TOP PRIORITIES

- [ ] ___________________
- [ ] ___________________

- [ ] ___________________
- [ ] ___________________

APPOINTMENTS & EVENTS

GET IN TOUCH WITH

- [ ] ___________________
- [ ] ___________________

MEALS

Breakfast

Lunch

Dinner

WEEKLY PLANNER

MONTH:

MONDAY

TUESDAY

WEDNESDAY

THURSDAY

FRIDAY

SATURDAY

SUNDAY

TO DO LIST

HABITS TRACKER

M T W T F S S

PERSONAL NOTES

MEAL PLANNER

WEEK: ———— MONTH: ————

MONDAY	B L D S

THIS WEEK'S GROCERY LIST

MONDAY
B
L
D
S

TUESDAY
B
L
D
S

WEDNESDAY
B
L
D
S

THURSDAY
B
L
D
S

FRIDAY
B
L
D
S

SATURDAY
B
L
D
S

SUNDAY
B
L
D
S

DAILY PLANNER

DATE: _______________ DAY: _______________

TO DO LIST

- [ ]
- [ ]
- [ ]
- [ ]
- [ ]
- [ ]
- [ ]

PERSONAL NOTES

TOP PRIORITIES

- [ ]
- [ ]

- [ ]
- [ ]

APPOINTMENTS & EVENTS

GET IN TOUCH WITH

- [ ]
- [ ]

MEALS

Breakfast

Lunch

Dinner

DAILY PLANNER

DATE: _______________ DAY: _______________

TO DO LIST

- [ ] ____________________
- [ ] ____________________
- [ ] ____________________
- [ ] ____________________
- [ ] ____________________
- [ ] ____________________
- [ ] ____________________

PERSONAL NOTES

TOP PRIORITIES

- [ ] ____________________
- [ ] ____________________

- [ ] ____________________
- [ ] ____________________

APPOINTMENTS & EVENTS

GET IN TOUCH WITH

- [ ] ____________________
- [ ] ____________________

MEALS

Breakfast

Lunch

Dinner

DAILY PLANNER

DATE: —————— DAY: ——————

TO DO LIST

PERSONAL NOTES

TOP PRIORITIES

APPOINTMENTS & EVENTS

GET IN TOUCH WITH

MEALS

Breakfast

Lunch

Dinner

DAILY PLANNER

DATE: ——————— DAY: ———————

TO DO LIST

- [ ]
- [ ]
- [ ]
- [ ]
- [ ]
- [ ]
- [ ]

PERSONAL NOTES

TOP PRIORITIES

- [ ]
- [ ]

- [ ]
- [ ]

APPOINTMENTS & EVENTS

GET IN TOUCH WITH

- [ ]
- [ ]

MEALS

Breakfast

Lunch

Dinner

DAILY PLANNER

DATE: _______ DAY: _______

TO DO LIST

- [ ] ____________________
- [ ] ____________________
- [ ] ____________________
- [ ] ____________________
- [ ] ____________________
- [ ] ____________________
- [ ] ____________________

PERSONAL NOTES

TOP PRIORITIES

- [ ] ____________________
- [ ] ____________________
- [ ] ____________________
- [ ] ____________________

APPOINTMENTS & EVENTS

GET IN TOUCH WITH

- [ ] ____________________
- [ ] ____________________

MEALS

Breakfast

Lunch

Dinner

DAILY PLANNER

DATE: ____________   DAY: ____________

TO DO LIST

☐ ______________________
☐ ______________________
☐ ______________________
☐ ______________________
☐ ______________________
☐ ______________________
☐ ______________________

PERSONAL NOTES

TOP PRIORITIES

☐ ______________________   ☐ ______________________
☐ ______________________   ☐ ______________________

APPOINTMENTS & EVENTS

GET IN TOUCH WITH

☐ ______________________
☐ ______________________

MEALS

Breakfast

Lunch

Dinner

DAILY PLANNER

DATE: _________ DAY: _________

TO DO LIST

- [ ] _______________________
- [ ] _______________________
- [ ] _______________________
- [ ] _______________________
- [ ] _______________________
- [ ] _______________________
- [ ] _______________________

PERSONAL NOTES

TOP PRIORITIES

- [ ] _______________________
- [ ] _______________________
- [ ] _______________________
- [ ] _______________________

APPOINTMENTS & EVENTS

GET IN TOUCH WITH

- [ ] _______________________
- [ ] _______________________

MEALS

Breakfast

Lunch

Dinner

WEEKLY PLANNER

MONTH:

MONDAY

TUESDAY

WEDNESDAY

THURSDAY

FRIDAY

SATURDAY

SUNDAY

TO DO LIST

HABITS TRACKER

M T W F S S

PERSONAL NOTES

MEAL PLANNER

WEEK: —————— MONTH: ——————

MONDAY
B
L
D
S

TUESDAY
B
L
D
S

WEDNESDAY
B
L
D
S

THURSDAY
B
L
D
S

FRIDAY
B
L
D
S

SATURDAY
B
L
D
S

SUNDAY
B
L
D
S

THIS WEEK'S GROCERY LIST

DAILY PLANNER

DATE: _______________ DAY: _______________

TO DO LIST

- ☐ _______________
- ☐ _______________
- ☐ _______________
- ☐ _______________
- ☐ _______________
- ☐ _______________
- ☐ _______________

PERSONAL NOTES

TOP PRIORITIES

- ☐ _______________
- ☐ _______________

- ☐ _______________
- ☐ _______________

APPOINTMENTS & EVENTS

GET IN TOUCH WITH

- ☐ _______________
- ☐ _______________

MEALS

Breakfast

Lunch

Dinner

DAILY PLANNER

DATE: ___________   DAY: ___________

TO DO LIST

PERSONAL NOTES

TOP PRIORITIES

APPOINTMENTS & EVENTS

GET IN TOUCH WITH

MEALS

Breakfast

Lunch

Dinner

DAILY PLANNER

DATE: ______________   DAY: ______________

TO DO LIST

PERSONAL NOTES

TOP PRIORITIES

APPOINTMENTS & EVENTS

GET IN TOUCH WITH

MEALS

Breakfast

Lunch

Dinner

DAILY PLANNER

DATE: ________________ DAY: ________________

TO DO LIST

- [ ] ________________
- [ ] ________________
- [ ] ________________
- [ ] ________________
- [ ] ________________
- [ ] ________________
- [ ] ________________

PERSONAL NOTES

TOP PRIORITIES

- [ ] ________________
- [ ] ________________

- [ ] ________________
- [ ] ________________

APPOINTMENTS & EVENTS

GET IN TOUCH WITH

- [ ] ________________
- [ ] ________________

MEALS

Breakfast

Lunch

Dinner

DAILY PLANNER

DATE: ___________ DAY: ___________

TO DO LIST

☐ ___________________________
☐ ___________________________
☐ ___________________________
☐ ___________________________
☐ ___________________________
☐ ___________________________
☐ ___________________________

PERSONAL NOTES

TOP PRIORITIES

☐ ___________________________
☐ ___________________________

☐ ___________________________
☐ ___________________________

APPOINTMENTS & EVENTS

GET IN TOUCH WITH

☐ ___________________________
☐ ___________________________

MEALS

Breakfast

Lunch

Dinner

DAILY PLANNER

DATE: _________________ DAY: _________________

TO DO LIST

☐ _______________________________
☐ _______________________________
☐ _______________________________
☐ _______________________________
☐ _______________________________
☐ _______________________________
☐ _______________________________

PERSONAL NOTES

TOP PRIORITIES

☐ _______________________________   ☐ _______________________________
☐ _______________________________   ☐ _______________________________

APPOINTMENTS & EVENTS

GET IN TOUCH WITH

☐ _______________________________
☐ _______________________________

MEALS

Breakfast

Lunch

Dinner

DAILY PLANNER

DATE: _____________ DAY: _____________

TO DO LIST

- ☐ _______________________
- ☐ _______________________
- ☐ _______________________
- ☐ _______________________
- ☐ _______________________
- ☐ _______________________
- ☐ _______________________

PERSONAL NOTES

TOP PRIORITIES

- ☐ _______________________
- ☐ _______________________

- ☐ _______________________
- ☐ _______________________

APPOINTMENTS & EVENTS

GET IN TOUCH WITH

- ☐ _______________________
- ☐ _______________________

MEALS

Breakfast

Lunch

Dinner

WEEKLY PLANNER

MONTH: _______________

MONDAY

TUESDAY

WEDNESDAY

THURSDAY

FRIDAY

SATURDAY

SUNDAY

TO DO LIST

☐ _______________

☐ _______________

☐ _______________

☐ _______________

☐ _______________

☐ _______________

☐ _______________

HABITS TRACKER

M T W T F S S

PERSONAL NOTES

MEAL PLANNER

WEEK: —————— MONTH: ——————

MONDAY
B
L
D
S

TUESDAY
B
L
D
S

WEDNESDAY
B
L
D
S

THURSDAY
B
L
D
S

FRIDAY
B
L
D
S

SATURDAY
B
L
D
S

SUNDAY
B
L
D
S

THIS WEEK'S GROCERY LIST

THIS WEEK'S GROCERY LIST

DAILY PLANNER

DATE: _______________ DAY: _______________

TO DO LIST

- ☐ _______________
- ☐ _______________
- ☐ _______________
- ☐ _______________
- ☐ _______________
- ☐ _______________
- ☐ _______________

TOP PRIORITIES

- ☐ _______________
- ☐ _______________

- ☐ _______________
- ☐ _______________

APPOINTMENTS & EVENTS

PERSONAL NOTES

GET IN TOUCH WITH

- ☐ _______________
- ☐ _______________

MEALS

Breakfast

Lunch

Dinner

DAILY PLANNER

DATE: ___________ DAY: ___________

TO DO LIST

- [ ] __________________________
- [ ] __________________________
- [ ] __________________________
- [ ] __________________________
- [ ] __________________________
- [ ] __________________________
- [ ] __________________________

PERSONAL NOTES

TOP PRIORITIES

- [ ] __________________________
- [ ] __________________________

- [ ] __________________________
- [ ] __________________________

APPOINTMENTS & EVENTS

GET IN TOUCH WITH

- [ ] __________________________
- [ ] __________________________

MEALS

Breakfast

Lunch

Dinner

DAILY PLANNER

DATE: _________ DAY: _________

TO DO LIST

- [ ]
- [ ]
- [ ]
- [ ]
- [ ]
- [ ]
- [ ]

PERSONAL NOTES

TOP PRIORITIES

- [ ]
- [ ]
- [ ]
- [ ]

APPOINTMENTS & EVENTS

GET IN TOUCH WITH

- [ ]
- [ ]

MEALS

Breakfast

Lunch

Dinner

DAILY PLANNER

DATE: ___________   DAY: ___________

TO DO LIST

- ☐ _______________
- ☐ _______________
- ☐ _______________
- ☐ _______________
- ☐ _______________
- ☐ _______________
- ☐ _______________

PERSONAL NOTES

TOP PRIORITIES

- ☐ _______________
- ☐ _______________

- ☐ _______________
- ☐ _______________

APPOINTMENTS & EVENTS

GET IN TOUCH WITH

- ☐ _______________
- ☐ _______________

MEALS

Breakfast

Lunch

Dinner

DAILY PLANNER

DATE: _____________   DAY: _____________

TO DO LIST

- ☐ _____________________
- ☐ _____________________
- ☐ _____________________
- ☐ _____________________
- ☐ _____________________
- ☐ _____________________
- ☐ _____________________

PERSONAL NOTES

TOP PRIORITIES

- ☐ _____________________
- ☐ _____________________

- ☐ _____________________
- ☐ _____________________

APPOINTMENTS & EVENTS

GET IN TOUCH WITH

- ☐ _____________________
- ☐ _____________________

MEALS

Breakfast

Lunch

Dinner

DAILY PLANNER

DATE: ———————   DAY: ———————

TO DO LIST

PERSONAL NOTES

TOP PRIORITIES

APPOINTMENTS & EVENTS

GET IN TOUCH WITH

MEALS

Breakfast

Lunch

Dinner

DAILY PLANNER

DATE: _________ DAY: _________

TO DO LIST

- ☐ _______________
- ☐ _______________
- ☐ _______________
- ☐ _______________
- ☐ _______________
- ☐ _______________
- ☐ _______________

PERSONAL NOTES

TOP PRIORITIES

- ☐ _______________
- ☐ _______________

- ☐ _______________
- ☐ _______________

APPOINTMENTS & EVENTS

GET IN TOUCH WITH

- ☐ _______________
- ☐ _______________

MEALS

Breakfast

Lunch

Dinner

WEEKLY PLANNER

MONTH:

MONDAY

TUESDAY

WEDNESDAY

THURSDAY

FRIDAY

SATURDAY

SUNDAY

TO DO LIST

HABITS TRACKER

M T W T F S S

PERSONAL NOTES

MEAL PLANNER

WEEK: —————— MONTH: ——————

MONDAY
B
L
D
S

TUESDAY
B
L
D
S

WEDNESDAY
B
L
D
S

THURSDAY
B
L
D
S

FRIDAY
B
L
D
S

SATURDAY
B
L
D
S

SUNDAY
B
L
D
S

THIS WEEK'S GROCERY LIST

FITNESS TRACKER

MONTH:

WEIGHT

105KG
95KG
85KG
75KG
65KG
55KG
45KG
35KG

JAN FEB MAR APR MAY JUN JUL AUG SEP OCT NOV DEC

MEASUREMENTS

	BUST	WAIST	HIPS	BUTT
JAN				
FEB				
MAR				
APR				
MAY				
JUN				
JUL				
AUG				
SEP				
OCT				
NOV				
DEC				

READING TRACKER

MONTH:

	TITLE	AUTHOR	GENRE	RATING
☐				☆ ☆ ☆ ☆ ☆
☐				☆ ☆ ☆ ☆ ☆
☐				☆ ☆ ☆ ☆ ☆
☐				☆ ☆ ☆ ☆ ☆
☐				☆ ☆ ☆ ☆ ☆
☐				☆ ☆ ☆ ☆ ☆
☐				☆ ☆ ☆ ☆ ☆
☐				☆ ☆ ☆ ☆ ☆
☐				☆ ☆ ☆ ☆ ☆
☐				☆ ☆ ☆ ☆ ☆
☐				☆ ☆ ☆ ☆ ☆
☐				☆ ☆ ☆ ☆ ☆

DAILY PLANNER

DATE: ______________   DAY: ______________

TO DO LIST

☐ ______________________________
☐ ______________________________
☐ ______________________________
☐ ______________________________
☐ ______________________________
☐ ______________________________
☐ ______________________________

PERSONAL NOTES

TOP PRIORITIES

☐ ______________________   ☐ ______________________
☐ ______________________   ☐ ______________________

APPOINTMENTS & EVENTS

GET IN TOUCH WITH

☐ ______________________________
☐ ______________________________

MEALS

Breakfast

Lunch

Dinner

DAILY PLANNER

DATE: _______________ DAY: _______________

TO DO LIST

- [ ]
- [ ]
- [ ]
- [ ]
- [ ]
- [ ]
- [ ]

PERSONAL NOTES

TOP PRIORITIES

- [ ]
- [ ]
- [ ]
- [ ]

APPOINTMENTS & EVENTS

GET IN TOUCH WITH

- [ ]
- [ ]

MEALS

Breakfast

Lunch

Dinner

DAILY PLANNER

DATE: _____________   DAY: _____________

TO DO LIST

PERSONAL NOTES

TOP PRIORITIES

APPOINTMENTS & EVENTS

GET IN TOUCH WITH

MEALS

Breakfast

Lunch

Dinner

DAILY PLANNER

DATE: ———————— DAY: ————————

TO DO LIST

- [ ]
- [ ]
- [ ]
- [ ]
- [ ]
- [ ]
- [ ]

PERSONAL NOTES

TOP PRIORITIES

- [ ]
- [ ]

- [ ]
- [ ]

APPOINTMENTS & EVENTS

GET IN TOUCH WITH

- [ ]
- [ ]

MEALS

Breakfast

Lunch

Dinner

DAILY PLANNER

DATE: _______________ DAY: _______________

TO DO LIST

PERSONAL NOTES

TOP PRIORITIES

APPOINTMENTS & EVENTS

GET IN TOUCH WITH

MEALS

Breakfast

Lunch

Dinner

DAILY PLANNER

DATE: ___________ DAY: ___________

TO DO LIST

- [ ] _______________
- [ ] _______________
- [ ] _______________
- [ ] _______________
- [ ] _______________
- [ ] _______________
- [ ] _______________

PERSONAL NOTES

TOP PRIORITIES

- [ ] _______________
- [ ] _______________
- [ ] _______________
- [ ] _______________

APPOINTMENTS & EVENTS

GET IN TOUCH WITH

- [ ] _______________
- [ ] _______________

MEALS

Breakfast

Lunch

Dinner

DAILY PLANNER

DATE: ______________   DAY: ______________

TO DO LIST

- ☐ __________________________
- ☐ __________________________
- ☐ __________________________
- ☐ __________________________
- ☐ __________________________
- ☐ __________________________
- ☐ __________________________

PERSONAL NOTES

TOP PRIORITIES

- ☐ __________________________
- ☐ __________________________

APPOINTMENTS & EVENTS

GET IN TOUCH WITH

- ☐ __________________________
- ☐ __________________________

MEALS

Breakfast

Lunch

Dinner

WEEKLY PLANNER

MONTH:

MONDAY

TUESDAY

WEDNESDAY

THURSDAY

FRIDAY

SATURDAY

SUNDAY

TO DO LIST

HABITS TRACKER

M T W T F S S

PERSONAL NOTES

MEAL PLANNER

WEEK: ———— MONTH: ————

MONDAY
B
L
D
S

TUESDAY
B
L
D
S

WEDNESDAY
B
L
D
S

THURSDAY
B
L
D
S

FRIDAY
B
L
D
S

SATURDAY
B
L
D
S

SUNDAY
B
L
D
S

THIS WEEK'S GROCERY LIST

THIS WEEK'S GROCERY LIST

DAILY PLANNER

DATE: ________________ DAY: ________________

TO DO LIST

- ☐ ________________
- ☐ ________________
- ☐ ________________
- ☐ ________________
- ☐ ________________
- ☐ ________________
- ☐ ________________

PERSONAL NOTES

TOP PRIORITIES

- ☐ ________________
- ☐ ________________

- ☐ ________________
- ☐ ________________

APPOINTMENTS & EVENTS

GET IN TOUCH WITH

- ☐ ________________
- ☐ ________________

MEALS

Breakfast

Lunch

Dinner

DAILY PLANNER

DATE: _______________ DAY: _______________

TO DO LIST

- [ ]
- [ ]
- [ ]
- [ ]
- [ ]
- [ ]
- [ ]

PERSONAL NOTES

TOP PRIORITIES

- [ ]
- [ ]
- [ ]
- [ ]

APPOINTMENTS & EVENTS

GET IN TOUCH WITH

- [ ]
- [ ]

MEALS

Breakfast

Lunch

Dinner

DAILY PLANNER

DATE: ___________ DAY: ___________

TO DO LIST

- [ ] ___________________________
- [ ] ___________________________
- [ ] ___________________________
- [ ] ___________________________
- [ ] ___________________________
- [ ] ___________________________
- [ ] ___________________________

PERSONAL NOTES

TOP PRIORITIES

- [ ] ___________________________
- [ ] ___________________________

- [ ] ___________________________
- [ ] ___________________________

APPOINTMENTS & EVENTS

GET IN TOUCH WITH

- [ ] ___________________________
- [ ] ___________________________

MEALS

Breakfast

Lunch

Dinner

DAILY PLANNER

DATE: ———————   DAY: ———————

TO DO LIST

- [ ] ______________________
- [ ] ______________________
- [ ] ______________________
- [ ] ______________________
- [ ] ______________________
- [ ] ______________________
- [ ] ______________________

PERSONAL NOTES

TOP PRIORITIES

- [ ] ______________________
- [ ] ______________________

- [ ] ______________________
- [ ] ______________________

APPOINTMENTS & EVENTS

GET IN TOUCH WITH

- [ ] ______________________
- [ ] ______________________

MEALS

Breakfast

Lunch

Dinner

DAILY PLANNER

DATE: ______________ DAY: ______________

TO DO LIST

- ☐ ____________________
- ☐ ____________________
- ☐ ____________________
- ☐ ____________________
- ☐ ____________________
- ☐ ____________________
- ☐ ____________________

PERSONAL NOTES

TOP PRIORITIES

- ☐ ____________________
- ☐ ____________________
- ☐ ____________________
- ☐ ____________________

APPOINTMENTS & EVENTS

GET IN TOUCH WITH

- ☐ ____________________
- ☐ ____________________

MEALS

Breakfast

Lunch

Dinner

DAILY PLANNER

DATE: —————— DAY: ——————

TO DO LIST

- ☐ ______________________
- ☐ ______________________
- ☐ ______________________
- ☐ ______________________
- ☐ ______________________
- ☐ ______________________
- ☐ ______________________

PERSONAL NOTES

TOP PRIORITIES

- ☐ ______________________
- ☐ ______________________
- ☐ ______________________
- ☐ ______________________

APPOINTMENTS & EVENTS

GET IN TOUCH WITH

- ☐ ______________________
- ☐ ______________________

MEALS

Breakfast

Lunch

Dinner

DAILY PLANNER

DATE: ——————— DAY: ———————

TO DO LIST

- ☐ ______________
- ☐ ______________
- ☐ ______________
- ☐ ______________
- ☐ ______________
- ☐ ______________
- ☐ ______________

TOP PRIORITIES

- ☐ ______________
- ☐ ______________
- ☐ ______________
- ☐ ______________

APPOINTMENTS & EVENTS

PERSONAL NOTES

GET IN TOUCH WITH

- ☐ ______________
- ☐ ______________

MEALS

Breakfast

Lunch

Dinner

WEEKLY PLANNER

MONTH:

MONDAY

TUESDAY

WEDNESDAY

THURSDAY

FRIDAY

SATURDAY

SUNDAY

TO DO LIST

HABITS TRACKER

M T W T F S S

PERSONAL NOTES

MEAL PLANNER

WEEK: ——————— MONTH: ———————

MONDAY
B
L
D
S

TUESDAY
B
L
D
S

WEDNESDAY
B
L
D
S

THURSDAY
B
L
D
S

FRIDAY
B
L
D
S

SATURDAY
B
L
D
S

SUNDAY
B
L
D
S

THIS WEEK'S GROCERY LIST

DAILY PLANNER

DATE: _______________ DAY: _______________

TO DO LIST

PERSONAL NOTES

TOP PRIORITIES

APPOINTMENTS & EVENTS

GET IN TOUCH WITH

MEALS

Breakfast

Lunch

Dinner

DAILY PLANNER

DATE: ___________ DAY: ___________

TO DO LIST

- [ ]
- [ ]
- [ ]
- [ ]
- [ ]
- [ ]
- [ ]

PERSONAL NOTES

TOP PRIORITIES

- [ ]
- [ ]
- [ ]
- [ ]

APPOINTMENTS & EVENTS

GET IN TOUCH WITH

- [ ]
- [ ]

MEALS

Breakfast

Lunch

Dinner

DAILY PLANNER

DATE: _________   DAY: _________

TO DO LIST

- ☐ _______________________
- ☐ _______________________
- ☐ _______________________
- ☐ _______________________
- ☐ _______________________
- ☐ _______________________
- ☐ _______________________

PERSONAL NOTES

TOP PRIORITIES

- ☐ _______________________
- ☐ _______________________

- ☐ _______________________
- ☐ _______________________

APPOINTMENTS & EVENTS

GET IN TOUCH WITH

- ☐ _______________________
- ☐ _______________________

MEALS

Breakfast

Lunch

Dinner

DAILY PLANNER

DATE: _________ DAY: _________

TO DO LIST

☐ __________________
☐ __________________
☐ __________________
☐ __________________
☐ __________________
☐ __________________
☐ __________________

PERSONAL NOTES

TOP PRIORITIES

☐ __________________   ☐ __________________
☐ __________________   ☐ __________________

APPOINTMENTS & EVENTS

GET IN TOUCH WITH

☐ __________________
☐ __________________

MEALS

Breakfast

Lunch

Dinner

DAILY PLANNER

DATE: __________ DAY: __________

TO DO LIST

- ☐ ______________________
- ☐ ______________________
- ☐ ______________________
- ☐ ______________________
- ☐ ______________________
- ☐ ______________________
- ☐ ______________________

PERSONAL NOTES

TOP PRIORITIES

- ☐ ______________________
- ☐ ______________________

- ☐ ______________________
- ☐ ______________________

APPOINTMENTS & EVENTS

GET IN TOUCH WITH

- ☐ ______________________
- ☐ ______________________

MEALS

Breakfast

Lunch

Dinner

DAILY PLANNER

DATE: —————— DAY: ——————

TO DO LIST

- ☐ ________________
- ☐ ________________
- ☐ ________________
- ☐ ________________
- ☐ ________________
- ☐ ________________
- ☐ ________________

PERSONAL NOTES

TOP PRIORITIES

- ☐ ________________
- ☐ ________________

- ☐ ________________
- ☐ ________________

APPOINTMENTS & EVENTS

GET IN TOUCH WITH

- ☐ ________________
- ☐ ________________

MEALS

Breakfast

Lunch

Dinner

DAILY PLANNER

DATE: _____________ DAY: _____________

TO DO LIST

PERSONAL NOTES

TOP PRIORITIES

APPOINTMENTS & EVENTS

GET IN TOUCH WITH

MEALS

Breakfast

Lunch

Dinner

WEEKLY PLANNER

MONTH:

MONDAY

TUESDAY

WEDNESDAY

THURSDAY

FRIDAY

SATURDAY

SUNDAY

TO DO LIST

- [ ]
- [ ]
- [ ]
- [ ]
- [ ]
- [ ]
- [ ]

HABITS TRACKER

M T W T F S S

PERSONAL NOTES

MEAL PLANNER

WEEK: ________ MONTH: ________

MONDAY
B
L
D
S

TUESDAY
B
L
D
S

WEDNESDAY
B
L
D
S

THURSDAY
B
L
D
S

FRIDAY
B
L
D
S

SATURDAY
B
L
D
S

SUNDAY
B
L
D
S

THIS WEEK'S GROCERY LIST

DAILY PLANNER

DATE: _______________ DAY: _______________

TO DO LIST

☐ _______________
☐ _______________
☐ _______________
☐ _______________
☐ _______________
☐ _______________
☐ _______________

PERSONAL NOTES

TOP PRIORITIES

☐ _______________   ☐ _______________
☐ _______________   ☐ _______________

APPOINTMENTS & EVENTS

GET IN TOUCH WITH

☐ _______________
☐ _______________

MEALS

Breakfast

Lunch

Dinner

DAILY PLANNER

DATE: _______ DAY: _______

TO DO LIST

- ☐ _______
- ☐ _______
- ☐ _______
- ☐ _______
- ☐ _______
- ☐ _______
- ☐ _______

PERSONAL NOTES

TOP PRIORITIES

- ☐ _______
- ☐ _______
- ☐ _______
- ☐ _______

APPOINTMENTS & EVENTS

GET IN TOUCH WITH

- ☐ _______
- ☐ _______

MEALS

Breakfast

Lunch

Dinner

DAILY PLANNER

DATE: ________ DAY: ________

TO DO LIST

- ☐ ____________________
- ☐ ____________________
- ☐ ____________________
- ☐ ____________________
- ☐ ____________________
- ☐ ____________________
- ☐ ____________________

PERSONAL NOTES

TOP PRIORITIES

- ☐ ____________________
- ☐ ____________________
- ☐ ____________________
- ☐ ____________________

APPOINTMENTS & EVENTS

GET IN TOUCH WITH

- ☐ ____________________
- ☐ ____________________

MEALS

Breakfast

Lunch

Dinner

DAILY PLANNER

DATE: _______ DAY: _______

TO DO LIST

- [ ] _______________
- [ ] _______________
- [ ] _______________
- [ ] _______________
- [ ] _______________
- [ ] _______________
- [ ] _______________

PERSONAL NOTES

TOP PRIORITIES

- [ ] _______________
- [ ] _______________

APPOINTMENTS & EVENTS

GET IN TOUCH WITH

- [ ] _______________
- [ ] _______________

MEALS

Breakfast

Lunch

Dinner

DAILY PLANNER

DATE: _____________   DAY: _____________

TO DO LIST

- [ ]
- [ ]
- [ ]
- [ ]
- [ ]
- [ ]
- [ ]

PERSONAL NOTES

TOP PRIORITIES

- [ ]
- [ ]
- [ ]
- [ ]

APPOINTMENTS & EVENTS

GET IN TOUCH WITH

- [ ]
- [ ]

MEALS

Breakfast

Lunch

Dinner

DAILY PLANNER

DATE: __________ DAY: __________

TO DO LIST

- ☐ ______________________
- ☐ ______________________
- ☐ ______________________
- ☐ ______________________
- ☐ ______________________
- ☐ ______________________
- ☐ ______________________

PERSONAL NOTES

TOP PRIORITIES

- ☐ ______________________
- ☐ ______________________
- ☐ ______________________
- ☐ ______________________

APPOINTMENTS & EVENTS

GET IN TOUCH WITH

- ☐ ______________________
- ☐ ______________________

MEALS

Breakfast

Lunch

Dinner

DAILY PLANNER

DATE: ————— DAY: —————

TO DO LIST

PERSONAL NOTES

TOP PRIORITIES

APPOINTMENTS & EVENTS

GET IN TOUCH WITH

MEALS

Breakfast

Lunch

Dinner

WEEKLY PLANNER

MONTH:

MONDAY

TUESDAY

WEDNESDAY

THURSDAY

FRIDAY

SATURDAY

SUNDAY

TO DO LIST

HABITS TRACKER

M T W T F S S

PERSONAL NOTES

MEAL PLANNER

WEEK: ———— MONTH: ————

MONDAY
B
L
D
S

TUESDAY
B
L
D
S

WEDNESDAY
B
L
D
S

THURSDAY
B
L
D
S

FRIDAY
B
L
D
S

SATURDAY
B
L
D
S

SUNDAY
B
L
D
S

THIS WEEK'S GROCERY LIST

MONTH: _______

MEASUREMENTS

	BUST	WAIST	HIPS	BUTT
JAN				
FEB				
MAR				
APR				
MAY				
JUN				
JUL				
AUG				
SEP				
OCT				
NOV				
DEC				

FITNESS TRACKER

WEIGHT

105KG
95KG
85KG
75KG
65KG
55KG
45KG
35KG

JAN FEB MAR APR MAY JUN JUL AUG SEP OCT NOV DEC

READING TRACKER

MONTH:

	TITLE	AUTHOR	GENRE	RATING
☐				☆ ☆ ☆ ☆ ☆
☐				☆ ☆ ☆ ☆ ☆
☐				☆ ☆ ☆ ☆ ☆
☐				☆ ☆ ☆ ☆ ☆
☐				☆ ☆ ☆ ☆ ☆
☐				☆ ☆ ☆ ☆ ☆
☐				☆ ☆ ☆ ☆ ☆
☐				☆ ☆ ☆ ☆ ☆
☐				☆ ☆ ☆ ☆ ☆
☐				☆ ☆ ☆ ☆ ☆
☐				☆ ☆ ☆ ☆ ☆
☐				☆ ☆ ☆ ☆ ☆

DAILY PLANNER

DATE: ______________ DAY: ______________

TO DO LIST

PERSONAL NOTES

TOP PRIORITIES

APPOINTMENTS & EVENTS

GET IN TOUCH WITH

MEALS

Breakfast

Lunch

Dinner

DAILY PLANNER

DATE: ———————— DAY: ————————

TO DO LIST

- [ ] ________________
- [ ] ________________
- [ ] ________________
- [ ] ________________
- [ ] ________________
- [ ] ________________
- [ ] ________________

PERSONAL NOTES

TOP PRIORITIES

- [ ] ________________
- [ ] ________________
- [ ] ________________
- [ ] ________________

APPOINTMENTS & EVENTS

GET IN TOUCH WITH

- [ ] ________________
- [ ] ________________

MEALS

Breakfast

Lunch

Dinner

DAILY PLANNER

DATE: _______   DAY: _______

TO DO LIST

- ☐ _______________________
- ☐ _______________________
- ☐ _______________________
- ☐ _______________________
- ☐ _______________________
- ☐ _______________________
- ☐ _______________________

PERSONAL NOTES

TOP PRIORITIES

- ☐ _______________________
- ☐ _______________________

- ☐ _______________________
- ☐ _______________________

APPOINTMENTS & EVENTS

GET IN TOUCH WITH

- ☐ _______________________
- ☐ _______________________

MEALS

Breakfast

Lunch

Dinner

DAILY PLANNER

DATE: ______________ DAY: ______________

TO DO LIST

- ☐ ________________________
- ☐ ________________________
- ☐ ________________________
- ☐ ________________________
- ☐ ________________________
- ☐ ________________________
- ☐ ________________________

PERSONAL NOTES

TOP PRIORITIES

- ☐ ________________________
- ☐ ________________________

- ☐ ________________________
- ☐ ________________________

APPOINTMENTS & EVENTS

GET IN TOUCH WITH

- ☐ ________________________
- ☐ ________________________

MEALS

Breakfast

Lunch

Dinner

DAILY PLANNER

DATE: _______________ DAY: _______________

TO DO LIST

☐ _______________
☐ _______________
☐ _______________
☐ _______________
☐ _______________
☐ _______________
☐ _______________

PERSONAL NOTES

TOP PRIORITIES

☐ _______________   ☐ _______________
☐ _______________   ☐ _______________

APPOINTMENTS & EVENTS

GET IN TOUCH WITH

☐ _______________
☐ _______________

MEALS

Breakfast

Lunch

Dinner

DAILY PLANNER

DATE: ——————— DAY: ———————

TO DO LIST

PERSONAL NOTES

TOP PRIORITIES

APPOINTMENTS & EVENTS

GET IN TOUCH WITH

MEALS

Breakfast

Lunch

Dinner

DAILY PLANNER

DATE: _______________ DAY: _______________

TO DO LIST

PERSONAL NOTES

TOP PRIORITIES

APPOINTMENTS & EVENTS

GET IN TOUCH WITH

MEALS

Breakfast

Lunch

Dinner

WEEKLY PLANNER

MONTH: ______________

MONDAY

TUESDAY

WEDNESDAY

THURSDAY

FRIDAY

SATURDAY

SUNDAY

TO DO LIST

- ☐ ______________
- ☐ ______________
- ☐ ______________
- ☐ ______________
- ☐ ______________
- ☐ ______________
- ☐ ______________

HABITS TRACKER

M T W T F S S

PERSONAL NOTES

MEAL PLANNER

WEEK: ——————— MONTH: ———————

MONDAY
B
L
D
S

TUESDAY
B
L
D
S

WEDNESDAY
B
L
D
S

THURSDAY
B
L
D
S

FRIDAY
B
L
D
S

SATURDAY
B
L
D
S

SUNDAY
B
L
D
S

THIS WEEK'S GROCERY LIST

DAILY PLANNER

DATE: ——————   DAY: ——————

TO DO LIST

PERSONAL NOTES

TOP PRIORITIES

APPOINTMENTS & EVENTS

GET IN TOUCH WITH

MEALS

Breakfast

Lunch

Dinner

DAILY PLANNER

DATE: _______________ DAY: _______________

TO DO LIST

- [ ] _______________
- [ ] _______________
- [ ] _______________
- [ ] _______________
- [ ] _______________
- [ ] _______________
- [ ] _______________

PERSONAL NOTES

TOP PRIORITIES

- [ ] _______________
- [ ] _______________

- [ ] _______________
- [ ] _______________

APPOINTMENTS & EVENTS

GET IN TOUCH WITH

- [ ] _______________
- [ ] _______________

MEALS

Breakfast

Lunch

Dinner

DAILY PLANNER

DATE: DAY:

TO DO LIST

PERSONAL NOTES

TOP PRIORITIES

APPOINTMENTS & EVENTS

GET IN TOUCH WITH

MEALS

Breakfast

Lunch

Dinner

DAILY PLANNER

DATE: __________ DAY: __________

TO DO LIST

PERSONAL NOTES

TOP PRIORITIES

APPOINTMENTS & EVENTS

GET IN TOUCH WITH

MEALS

Breakfast

Lunch

Dinner

DAILY PLANNER

DATE: —————————— DAY: ——————————

TO DO LIST

PERSONAL NOTES

TOP PRIORITIES

APPOINTMENTS & EVENTS

GET IN TOUCH WITH

MEALS

Breakfast

Lunch

Dinner

DAILY PLANNER

DATE: ______________ DAY: ______________

TO DO LIST

PERSONAL NOTES

TOP PRIORITIES

APPOINTMENTS & EVENTS

GET IN TOUCH WITH

MEALS

Breakfast

Lunch

Dinner

DAILY PLANNER

DATE: —————— DAY: ——————

TO DO LIST

- ☐ ______________________
- ☐ ______________________
- ☐ ______________________
- ☐ ______________________
- ☐ ______________________
- ☐ ______________________
- ☐ ______________________

PERSONAL NOTES

TOP PRIORITIES

- ☐ ______________________
- ☐ ______________________
- ☐ ______________________
- ☐ ______________________

APPOINTMENTS & EVENTS

GET IN TOUCH WITH

- ☐ ______________________
- ☐ ______________________

MEALS

Breakfast

Lunch

Dinner

WEEKLY PLANNER

MONTH:

MONDAY

TUESDAY

WEDNESDAY

THURSDAY

FRIDAY

SATURDAY

SUNDAY

TO DO LIST

HABITS TRACKER

M T W T F S S

PERSONAL NOTES

MEAL PLANNER

WEEK: —————— MONTH: ——————

MONDAY
B
L
D
S

TUESDAY
B
L
D
S

WEDNESDAY
B
L
D
S

THURSDAY
B
L
D
S

FRIDAY
B
L
D
S

SATURDAY
B
L
D
S

SUNDAY
B
L
D
S

THIS WEEK'S GROCERY LIST

DAILY PLANNER

DATE: _________ DAY: _________

TO DO LIST

PERSONAL NOTES

TOP PRIORITIES

APPOINTMENTS & EVENTS

GET IN TOUCH WITH

MEALS

Breakfast

Lunch

Dinner

DAILY PLANNER

DATE: —————— DAY: ——————

TO DO LIST

- ☐ ——————————
- ☐ ——————————
- ☐ ——————————
- ☐ ——————————
- ☐ ——————————
- ☐ ——————————
- ☐ ——————————

PERSONAL NOTES

TOP PRIORITIES

- ☐ ——————————
- ☐ ——————————
- ☐ ——————————
- ☐ ——————————

APPOINTMENTS & EVENTS

GET IN TOUCH WITH

- ☐ ——————————
- ☐ ——————————

MEALS

Breakfast

Lunch

Dinner

DAILY PLANNER

DATE: ______________   DAY: ______________

TO DO LIST

- ☐ ___________________
- ☐ ___________________
- ☐ ___________________
- ☐ ___________________
- ☐ ___________________
- ☐ ___________________
- ☐ ___________________

PERSONAL NOTES

TOP PRIORITIES

- ☐ ___________________
- ☐ ___________________

- ☐ ___________________
- ☐ ___________________

APPOINTMENTS & EVENTS

GET IN TOUCH WITH

- ☐ ___________________
- ☐ ___________________

MEALS

Breakfast

Lunch

Dinner

DAILY PLANNER

DATE: _____________ DAY: _____________

TO DO LIST

PERSONAL NOTES

TOP PRIORITIES

APPOINTMENTS & EVENTS

GET IN TOUCH WITH

MEALS

Breakfast

Lunch

Dinner

DAILY PLANNER

DATE: _______________ DAY: _______________

TO DO LIST

- [ ] _______________
- [ ] _______________
- [ ] _______________
- [ ] _______________
- [ ] _______________
- [ ] _______________
- [ ] _______________

PERSONAL NOTES

TOP PRIORITIES

- [ ] _______________
- [ ] _______________

- [ ] _______________
- [ ] _______________

APPOINTMENTS & EVENTS

GET IN TOUCH WITH

- [ ] _______________
- [ ] _______________

MEALS

Breakfast

Lunch

Dinner

DAILY PLANNER

DATE: __________   DAY: __________

TO DO LIST

- ☐ __________________________
- ☐ __________________________
- ☐ __________________________
- ☐ __________________________
- ☐ __________________________
- ☐ __________________________
- ☐ __________________________

PERSONAL NOTES

TOP PRIORITIES

- ☐ __________________________
- ☐ __________________________
- ☐ __________________________
- ☐ __________________________

APPOINTMENTS & EVENTS

GET IN TOUCH WITH

- ☐ __________________________
- ☐ __________________________

MEALS

Breakfast

Lunch

Dinner

DAILY PLANNER

DATE: ________ DAY: ________

TO DO LIST

- [ ] ________
- [ ] ________
- [ ] ________
- [ ] ________
- [ ] ________
- [ ] ________
- [ ] ________

PERSONAL NOTES

TOP PRIORITIES

- [ ] ________
- [ ] ________
- [ ] ________
- [ ] ________

APPOINTMENTS & EVENTS

GET IN TOUCH WITH

- [ ] ________
- [ ] ________

MEALS

Breakfast

Lunch

Dinner

WEEKLY PLANNER

MONTH:

MONDAY

TUESDAY

WEDNESDAY

THURSDAY

FRIDAY

SATURDAY

SUNDAY

TO DO LIST

HABITS TRACKER

M T W T F S S

PERSONAL NOTES

MEAL PLANNER

WEEK: ———————— MONTH: ————————

MONDAY
B
L
D
S

TUESDAY
B
L
D
S

WEDNESDAY
B
L
D
S

THURSDAY
B
L
D
S

FRIDAY
B
L
D
S

SATURDAY
B
L
D
S

SUNDAY
B
L
D
S

THIS WEEK'S GROCERY LIST

DAILY PLANNER

DATE: _________ DAY: _________

TO DO LIST

- ☐ _______________________
- ☐ _______________________
- ☐ _______________________
- ☐ _______________________
- ☐ _______________________
- ☐ _______________________
- ☐ _______________________

PERSONAL NOTES

TOP PRIORITIES

- ☐ _______________________
- ☐ _______________________
- ☐ _______________________
- ☐ _______________________

APPOINTMENTS & EVENTS

GET IN TOUCH WITH

- ☐ _______________________
- ☐ _______________________

MEALS

Breakfast

Lunch

Dinner

DAILY PLANNER

DATE: ————————   DAY: ————————

TO DO LIST

☐ ________________________
☐ ________________________
☐ ________________________
☐ ________________________
☐ ________________________
☐ ________________________
☐ ________________________

PERSONAL NOTES

TOP PRIORITIES

☐ ________________   ☐ ________________
☐ ________________   ☐ ________________

APPOINTMENTS & EVENTS

GET IN TOUCH WITH

☐ ________________________
☐ ________________________

MEALS

Breakfast

Lunch

Dinner

DAILY PLANNER

DATE: ______________ DAY: ______________

TO DO LIST

PERSONAL NOTES

TOP PRIORITIES

APPOINTMENTS & EVENTS

GET IN TOUCH WITH

MEALS

Breakfast

Lunch

Dinner

DAILY PLANNER

DATE: ___________   DAY: ___________

TO DO LIST

- [ ] ________________
- [ ] ________________
- [ ] ________________
- [ ] ________________
- [ ] ________________
- [ ] ________________
- [ ] ________________

PERSONAL NOTES

TOP PRIORITIES

- [ ] ________________
- [ ] ________________
- [ ] ________________
- [ ] ________________

APPOINTMENTS & EVENTS

GET IN TOUCH WITH

- [ ] ________________
- [ ] ________________

MEALS

Breakfast

Lunch

Dinner

DAILY PLANNER

DATE: _________________ DAY: _________________

TO DO LIST

- [ ] _______________________
- [ ] _______________________
- [ ] _______________________
- [ ] _______________________
- [ ] _______________________
- [ ] _______________________
- [ ] _______________________

PERSONAL NOTES

TOP PRIORITIES

- [ ] _______________________
- [ ] _______________________

- [ ] _______________________
- [ ] _______________________

APPOINTMENTS & EVENTS

GET IN TOUCH WITH

- [ ] _______________________
- [ ] _______________________

MEALS

Breakfast

Lunch

Dinner

DAILY PLANNER

DATE: ———————— DAY: ————————

TO DO LIST

PERSONAL NOTES

TOP PRIORITIES

APPOINTMENTS & EVENTS

GET IN TOUCH WITH

MEALS

Breakfast

Lunch

Dinner

DAILY PLANNER

DATE: ______________   DAY: ______________

TO DO LIST

- ☐ ______________
- ☐ ______________
- ☐ ______________
- ☐ ______________
- ☐ ______________
- ☐ ______________
- ☐ ______________

PERSONAL NOTES

TOP PRIORITIES

- ☐ ______________
- ☐ ______________
- ☐ ______________
- ☐ ______________

APPOINTMENTS & EVENTS

GET IN TOUCH WITH

- ☐ ______________
- ☐ ______________

MEALS

Breakfast

Lunch

Dinner

WEEKLY PLANNER

MONTH: _______________

MONDAY

TUESDAY

WEDNESDAY

THURSDAY

FRIDAY

SATURDAY

SUNDAY

TO DO LIST

HABITS TRACKER

M T W T F S S

PERSONAL NOTES

MEAL PLANNER

WEEK: ———— MONTH: ————

MONDAY
B
L
D
S

TUESDAY
B
L
D
S

WEDNESDAY
B
L
D
S

THURSDAY
B
L
D
S

FRIDAY
B
L
D
S

SATURDAY
B
L
D
S

SUNDAY
B
L
D
S

THIS WEEK'S GROCERY LIST

FITNESS TRACKER

MONTH: _______________

WEIGHT

105KG
95KG
85KG
75KG
65KG
55KG
45KG
35KG

JAN FEB MAR APR MAY JUN JUL AUG SEP OCT NOV DEC

MEASUREMENTS

	BUST	WAIST	HIPS	BUTT
JAN				
FEB				
MAR				
APR				
MAY				
JUN				
JUL				
AUG				
SEP				
OCT				
NOV				
DEC				

READING TRACKER

MONTH: ______________

	TITLE	AUTHOR	GENRE	RATING
☐				☆ ☆ ☆ ☆ ☆
☐				☆ ☆ ☆ ☆ ☆
☐				☆ ☆ ☆ ☆ ☆
☐				☆ ☆ ☆ ☆ ☆
☐				☆ ☆ ☆ ☆ ☆
☐				☆ ☆ ☆ ☆ ☆
☐				☆ ☆ ☆ ☆ ☆
☐				☆ ☆ ☆ ☆ ☆
☐				☆ ☆ ☆ ☆ ☆
☐				☆ ☆ ☆ ☆ ☆
☐				☆ ☆ ☆ ☆ ☆
☐				☆ ☆ ☆ ☆ ☆

JOURNAL

DATE: __________   DAY: __________

JOURNAL

DATE: _____________ DAY: _____________

JOURNAL

DATE: _____________ DAY: _____________

JOURNAL

DATE: —————— DAY: ——————

JOURNAL

DATE: ————— DAY: —————

JOURNAL

DATE: _____________ DAY: _____________